THE LECTIN DIET
FOOD LIST

BY THE LECTIN HEROES

Copyright: The Lectin Heroes 2021

All rights reserved. No part of this guide may be reproduced in any form without permission in writing from the publisher except in the case of brief quotations embodied in critical articles or reviews.

LEGAL & DISCLAIMER

The information contained in this book is not designed to replace or take the place of any form of medicine or professional medical advice. The information in this book has been provided for educational and entertainment purposes only.

You need to consult a professional medical practitioner in order to ensure you are both healthy enough and able to make use of this information. Always consult your professional medical practitioner before undertaking any new dietary regime, and particularly after reading this book.

The information contained in this book has been compiled from sources deemed reliable, and it is accurate to the best of the Author's knowledge; however, the Author cannot guarantee its accuracy and validity and cannot be held liable for any errors or omissions.

You must consult your doctor or get professional medical advice before using any suggested information in this book.

Upon using the information contained in this book, you agree to hold harmless the Author, and Publisher, from and against any damages, costs, and expenses, including any legal fees potentially resulting from the application of any of the information provided by this guide. This disclaimer applies to any damages or injury caused by the use and application, whether directly or indirectly, of any advice or information presented, whether for breach of contract, tort, negligence, personal injury, criminal intent, or under any other cause of action. You agree to accept all risks of using the information presented inside this book.

INTRODUCTION

Congratulations on choosing this book. We wrote it because we suffer from food intolerances and sensitivities ourselves, and we were frustrated at how so much information out there seems to confuse us and conflict with other sources.

Essentially, many of the top lectin resources disagree with each other. Which is not very helpful. One will tell you something is low-lectin, and another high-lectin.

So we decided to take the world's best and most trusted lectin guides and compile the information into one easy-to-consult food list.

Trust us, it's been quite the process.

Even as we wrote this guide, we noticed that many of the top lists massively disagree on lectin content in food.

WHAT EVEN ARE LECTINS?

Lectins are proteins that bind to carbohydrates and can be found in all plants as a defence mechanism. When consumed, they may cause problems as it's difficult for the gut to break down lectins. As the proteins bind onto cells for a long period of time, it's thought that they can cause an autoimmune response (source: *Harvard T.H. Chan School of Public Health*).

As we know now, that's the nature of lectin content and issues. Everybody reacts differently, and foods even show up differently depending on the amount of lectins present and the type of carbohydrates that binds them.

That's why we wanted to write this list. We believe it is the most comprehensive out there, and where there is debate, we have deferred to many of these top sources. With all that said, there will be areas you disagree on and that is why a) approach any new food with caution, and b) always consult your medical practitioner before making any dietary changes.

We know this list will never be definitive, and we will continue to refine it as more information becomes available. But it means you must approach every food cautiously.

We're not going to chew over the reasons behind your lectin issues. You've almost certainly done your research on it, and that's why you are here in the first place, for the most comprehensive low-lectin food list available.

If you are sensitive to lectins, no matter what kind, use this book to avoid foods that are high in lectin content. These can include major culprits like beans, lentils, peas, soybeans, peanuts and wheat. As we will also remind you throughout the book, it's possible to reduce lectins in food by soaking, cooking and sprouting.

So you'll learn all about what to avoid from this book, and you might start to feel a lot better from your lectin issues.

It's also important to point out that not everybody needs to avoid lectins. Research conducted on active lectin consumption in humans and it's long-term health effects are very limited. However, certain groups of people e.g. those diagnosed with specific conditions have found eliminating lectins helped with digestive issues and inflammation.

All of which means you should consult with your practitioner to determine the correct course for you. Please keep in mind that materials and resources like this book are no substitute for medical advice and not intended as such.

Now, let's get straight onto the list.

HOW TO USE THIS FOOD LIST

This book works like a dictionary. Look for a food, drink or ingredient alphabetically or on search.

Once you find what you are looking for, it is scored between 1 and 5 for lectin levels based on careful analysis of the world's best sources (listed below) for lectin content.

Some online titles detail either cup size, serving size or precise amount of mg of lectins per 100 g. That can be really useful, but we're all different, and that means one of our servings might be three of somebody else's.

So we've made it more straightforward in this book. We've consulted those sites, and each food gets a score. The higher the score, the better it is for your low lectin diet.

- 5 is best (indicates foods that are the lowest in lectin as per our sources)

- 4 is good (still very low in lectin and still ok to consume on a low-lectin diet)

- 3 is moderate (indicates some lectins but test carefully)

- 2 is poor (a potentially poor choice and a food to test extremely cautiously)
- 1 is worst (indicates poor choice for a low-lectin diet, and one to avoid)

So on a low-lectin diet, you would look to consume more 5 foods and cutting out 1 foods.

As time goes on, with the help of a skilled practitioner, you would look to address the root cause of your lectin sensitivity and try an elimination-style diet to work out which foods are causing symptoms.

We decided on a scoring system between 1 and 5 as many food lists only group foods into 'high' or 'low' lectin (or 'bad' and 'good', and we feel there is considerably more nuance to food intolerances, allergies and analysis. Respected sites can disagree on major foods so we've tried to reflect that in our list.

At this point, we probably need to insert a disclaimer. Our aim is to learn more about which foods contain lectins, and live a healthy, balanced life in every aspect. This book has been a labour of love, but it has been a challenge to put together as the major lists disagree so often about lectin content.

Consult your doctor or get professional medical advice before using the information in this book. This is a guide, not a definitive list as everybody is individual.

Keep this book close by when you cook or eat out, and dip in and out whenever you need to check if something is low-lectin.

SOURCES

These excellent sources come highly recommended in your further research on lectins. As far as possible we have consulted all these sites in our research into this food list.

Please do click on these top lectin diet sites for further reading. We consider them to be the best sources out there.

- Harvard T.H. Chan School of Public Health - Lectins
  https://www.hsph.harvard.edu/nutritionsource/anti-nutrients/lectins/

- Precision Nutrition - All about lectins
  https://www.precisionnutrition.com/all-about-lectins

- Dietetically Speaking - The lectin-free diet
  https://dieteticallyspeaking.com/the-lectin-free-diet/

- Mental Food Chain - 400+ foods high in lectins and lectin-free food list https://www.mentalfoodchain.com/foods-high-in-lectins/

- Amos Institute - What are lectins and the lectin-free diet?
  https://amosinstitute.com/blog/what-are-lectins-and-the-lectin-free-diet/

- Mayo Clinic - What are dietary lectins and should you avoid eating them?
  https://amosinstitute.com/blog/what-are-lectins-and-the-lectin-free-diet/

- Everyday Health - Lectin-Free Diet: Benefits, Risks, Food Choices, and More
  https://www.everydayhealth.com/diet-nutrition/lectin-free-diet/

- Dr. Steven Gundry Diet Food List
  https://gundrymd.com/dr-gundry-diet-food-list/

- Restart Med - Food List
  https://www.restartmed.com/wp-content/uploads/2018/09/Foods-high-in-Lectins-1.pdf

- Pritikin Longevitiy Center + Spa - Are nightshade vegetables bad for you?
  https://www.pritikin.com/are-nightshade-vegetables-bad

- Shawn Wells - Your guide to lectins, phytates & oxalates
  https://shawnwells.com/2020/07/your-guide-to-lectins-phytates-oxalates/

- Daytona Wellness Center - What should you eat
  https://daytonawellnesscenter.com/what-should-you-eat-published-june-18-2017-by-dr-daniel-thomas-do-ms/

- Healthline - Everything you need to know about dietary lectins
  https://www.healthline.com/nutrition/dietary-lectins

- Eating Well - What is the lectin-free diet?
  https://www.eatingwell.com/article/7827647/what-is-the-lectin-free-diet/

- Mind Body Green - Foods high in lectins: what to avoid to heal your gut
  https://www.mindbodygreen.com/articles/foods-high-in-lectins

THE FOOD LIST

Acerola: 3

Acerola contains a lot of vitamin C. Having scoured the research we have found only limited information. Given that acerola is similar to cherries, it may be low in lectins.

Agave syrup: 1

Also known as agave nectar. Agave itself and agave syrup are thought to be high in lectins.

Alcohol: 3

Varies by alcohol. Check individual alcohols in list.

Beer should be avoided as it's thought to be high in lectins.

Red wine contains high levels of Polyphenols (antioxidants) compared to other types of wine (including white wine) however, it's thought to also contains lectins. Some experts permit drinking wine high in Polyphenols (in moderation) on a low-lectin diet. Test red wine carefully.

It's unclear whether sparkling wine, brandy, rum, spirits and schnapps should be avoided. Consume in moderation and test carefully. Dessert wines, sweet wines and white wines should also be avoided. Given the high sugar content, these wines also don't seem to have the same benefits as red wine.

Tequila is something that many seem to enjoy on a low-lectin diet, but again, test carefully.

Algae: 4

Thought to be low in lectins. Red algae should be avoided as these are high in lectins and often consumed raw.

Almond: 3

Almond skin is high in lectins.

Top tip to enjoy almonds: you can eat lower-lectin almonds by removing the skin and blanching them to lower the lectin content. Soaking and blanching will be your friend when it comes to living with lectin sensitivities.

Anchovies: 5

Low in lectins. Opt for wild caught anchovies as these are supposed to contain higher levels of omega-3s.

Apple: 5

Low in lectins. Best to consume when apple is in season. It's thought that fruits in season may contain less lectins than when they're out of season.

Note the high sugar content in apples. According to the US Department of Agriculture, a medium-sized apple contains approximately 19g of sugar.

Apple cider vinegar: 5

It's thought that all types of vinegar are allowed on a low-lectin diet.

You'll read about soaking and sprouting quite a bit in this book. To decrease lectin content in foods, "adding a tiny splash of apple cider vinegar to soaking water may help neutralise the lectins further" (source: Simply Nourished Nutrition).

Apricot: 5

Allowed on a low-lectin diet. Best to consume when apricot is in season.

Artichokes: 4

Contains relatively little lectin.

Artificial sweeteners: 2

Very little research on lectins in artificial sweeteners; however, these should be eliminated.

We suggest avoiding artificial sweeteners due to the potential negative effects on your gut microbiome.

Asparagus: 3

According to Healthline and Shawn Wells, asparagus contains relatively little lectin. Another source confirmed the lectins found in asparagus "whether cooked or consumed raw, do not appear to cause significant GI problems". Test carefully.

Aubergine: 1

Also called *eggplant*.

Part of the nightshade family which are thought to be high in lectins, particularly in the seeds and peels. So you could take the seeds and the peel off but still probably best avoided.

Avocado: 4

Full of nutrients, this superfood is thought to be low-lectin.

Bamboo shoots: 5

Thought to be low-lectin.

Note that bamboo shoots should never be consumed raw or unprocessed due to natural toxins present which may cause health problems

(Source: *Nongdam P, Tikendra L. The Nutritional Facts of Bamboo Shoots and Their Usage as Important Traditional Foods of Northeast India*).

Banana: 3

We've given banana a rating of 3 based on the fact that they vary massively by ripeness. Avoid ripe bananas. Instead, go for green bananas which are safe to eat on a low-lectin diet.

Studies have also shown that lectins from bananas become more potent after heating (source: *https://dadamo.com/txt/index.pl?1007*) therefore, cooking or baking bananas should also be avoided.

Barley: 1

High in lectins. One to put in your 'avoid' list.

Barley malt, malt: 1

Considered a whole grain. Avoid as high in lectins.

Basil: 5

Thought to be low-lectin.

Beans: 1

High in lectins (including borlotti beans, broad beans and green beans). One to put in your 'avoid' list.

If you want to consume beans, the FDA recommends boiling them for 30 minutes to reduce lectin content.

Avoid canned beans as most of these have not been soaked or cooked to reduce lectin content.

As previously reiterated, soaking may reduce lectin content.

Beef: 5

Beef may be consumed on a low-lectin diet.

Avoid corn-fed beef and opt for grass-fed instead for general health reasons.

Beer: 1

Avoid as it's thought to be high in lectins.

Beetroot: 5

Also known as *Beets*. These may be consumed on a low lectin diet.

Kimberly Gomer, Director of Nutrition at the Pritikin Longevity Center in Miami confirmed the lectins found in beets "whether cooked or consumed raw, do not appear to cause significant GI problems".

It's worth noting that the best way to retain the nutrients is to gently sautéed, steam or roast them (source: *Stacy Mitchell Doyle, M.D., founder of FoodTherapyMD.com*).

Also note that beetroot is very high in oxalate and therefore one to avoid if you have multiple food sensitivities.

Bell pepper (hot or sweet): 1

Part of the nightshade family which are high in lectins particularly in the seeds and peels.

Bison: 5

Thought to be low-lectin. Opt for grass-fed bison.

Bivalves (mussels, oyster, clams, scallops): 3

A study found lectins present in bivalves (source: *ResearchGate: Lectins with Varying Specificity and Biological Activity from Marine Bivalves*) however, we're not sure of the lectin levels. Having studied the limited available research we'd ask you to test carefully. (Who knew these seafoods were called bivalves?)

Black caraway: 2

It's unclear whether black caraway are high in lectins but we know that caraway seeds are a source of lectins (source: Functional Nutrition Library).

Blackberry: 3

Mixed opinion on this one, as with so much in the lectin world.

One source confirms blackberries are a source of lectins. In Nathan Sharon's book *Lectins*, he confirmed that blackberries *"exhibit lectin activity"*.

However, other sources disagree.

Best to consume when blackberries are in season (source: Health Canal). Test carefully.

Blackcurrants: 2

Also known as *currants*. Thought to be a source of lectins.

Blue cheeses: 3

Cheese acquires lectins from the moulds that grow within it (source: *Understanding Arthritis, The Clinical Way Forward by W. Fox, D. Freed*). Test carefully as moulds are used in blue cheese production.

Blue fenugreek: 3

Blue fenugreek has a milder, less bitter taste than normal fenugreek. There is a limited amount of lectin research on blue fenugreek, but there are lectins present in fenugreek (source: Food and Nutrition Journal).

Blueberries: 3

Mixed opinion. Some sources confirm that blueberries do not contain lectins whereas other sources say blueberries contain relatively little lectin.

Test carefully. As with all fruits, it's best to consume when blueberries are in season.

A study found *"a lack of the antinutrients lectins"* in Andean blueberries.

(source: *Baenas N, Ruales J, Moreno DA, Barrio DA, Stinco CM, Martínez-Cifuentes G, Meléndez-Martínez AJ, García-Ruiz A. Characterization of Andean Blueberry in Bioactive Compounds, Evaluation of Biological Properties, and In Vitro Bioaccessibility*)

Bok choi: 5

Sometimes also written as *bok choy*. A lovely leafy green veg. Try sautéing or lightly roasting for 15 minutes.

Falls under the cruciferous vegetable family (includes broccoli, kale, cabbage, radish etc.). These are thought to be low-lectin and rich in vitamin C, folate and fiber.

Borlotti beans: 1

High in lectins. One to put in your 'avoid' list.

If you want to consume beans, the FDA recommends boiling them for 30 minutes to reduce lectin content.

Avoid canned beans as most of these have not been soaked or cooked to reduce lectin content.

Bouillon: 3

Also known as *broth*.

Broth is made from simmering water with either meat, fish or seafood. It seems that the amount of lectins depends on the type of broth.

Shop-bought stocks and bouillons can have a lot of different ingredients, so it's always worth checking closely. Very difficult to give a rating as there's very little research after careful analysis. Test carefully.

Boysenberry: 3

A cross of loganberry, blackberry and raspberry. Given that loganberry, blackberry and raspberry all contain lectins, we think there are moderate amounts of lectin in boysenberries.

Brandy: 3

A distilled liquor made from fermented fruit juice or wine (source: Whiskey Bon). It's not clear-cut whether brandy should be avoided as brandy can be made from a range of fruits from grapes to pears, raspberries, apples, cherries etc. It seems that the lectin content could depend on the type of fruit used during the process.

As with all alcohol, consume in moderation and test carefully. Very difficult to give a rating.

Brazil nut: 5

Allowed on a low-lectin diet.

Bread: 1

High in lectins. One to put in your 'avoid' list.

Broad-leaved garlic: 4

Also known as *wild garlic*. Given that garlic is allowed on a low-lectin diet, broad-leaved garlic may be allowed too.

Broad beans: 1

Also known as *Vicia Faba*. These are high in lectins. One to put in your 'avoid' list.

If you want to consume beans, the FDA recommends boiling them for 30 minutes to reduce lectin content.

Avoid canned beans as most of these have not been soaked or cooked to reduce lectin content (source: The Woodlands Institute).

Broccoli: 5

Falls under the cruciferous vegetable family (includes Brussels sprouts, kale, cabbage, radish etc.).

These are thought to be low-lectin and rich in vitamin C, folate and fiber.

Brussels sprouts: 5

Falls under the cruciferous vegetable family (includes broccoli, kale, cabbage, radish etc.).

Again, these are thought to be low-lectin and rich in vitamin C, folate and fiber.

Buckwheat: 2

Lectins are present but the lectin content may be reduced by soaking, sprouting and fermenting the buckwheat (source: Irena Macri, Nutrition Coach).

Butter: 4

Not all butter is created equal.

We recommend opting for grass-fed butter due to the higher proportion of healthy fats. Grass-fed butter is also rich in Vitamin A which is necessary for normal vision, the immune system and reproduction (source: Healthline).

Then the whole subject of butter gets more complicated.

Butters made with A2 milk (from cows that originate in the Channel Islands and Southern France) are possibly better for a low-lectin diet (source: Claudia Curici, Author).

Avoid butter produced from A1 milk (regular milk with casein protein). We appreciate that it's difficult to know how shop bought milk is produced and suggest testing carefully.

Cabbage: 5

Falls under the cruciferous vegetable family (includes broccoli, kale, Brussel sprouts, radish etc.). These are thought to be your low-lectin friend.

Cactus pear: 5

Also known as *nopales*. It's thought that these may be consumed on a low-lectin diet.

According to Mayo Clinic, cactus pears are promoted for treating diabetes, high cholesterol, obesity and hangovers. Enjoy as part of a healthy diet.

Cardamom: 3

Seeds from the cardamon plant. A number of sources outline the benefits of cardamom and even call it *"the Queen Spices"*. A study found *"antibacterial and anti-inflammatory properties"* of cardamom against periodontal infections.

(source: *Souissi M, Azelmat J, Chaieb K, Grenier D. Antibacterial and anti-inflammatory activities of cardamom (Elettaria cardamomum) extracts: Potential therapeutic benefits for periodontal infections*)

Note that most seeds aren't allowed on a low-lectin diet but if due to the health benefits cardamom, you may want to consume. Test carefully.

Carrot: 5

Contain relatively little lectin.

Cashew nut: 1

High in lectins, but cooking helps reduce lectin content. Even so, still one to approach extremely cautiously.

Interesting side note: Did you know that raw cashew nuts are toxic? This is due to a chemical called urushiol contained in the shells and this is why cashew nuts sold in stores have been roasted or steamed before shelled (source: Medicine Net).

Cassava: 5

Cassava is thought to be fine to consume in limited quantities unless you have a pre-existing health condition.

Cassava flour is also lectin-free. According to Lectin Free Mama's blog, cassava flour "yields the fluffiest, most bread-like baked goods you can imagine". Why not try baking with cassava flour?

Cauliflower: 5

Falls under the cruciferous vegetable family (includes broccoli, kale, cabbage, radish etc.).

These are thought to be low-lectin and rich in vitamin C, folate and fiber.

Celery: 5

Good news, celery fans. Celery falls under the lowest lectin content options for a low-lectin diet.

Cep mushrooms: 5

Mushrooms are also thought to fall under the lowest lectin content options for a low-lectin diet.

Chamomile and chamomile tea: 5

Tea is thought to be a better choice for a low-lectin diet than coffee. It's thought that tea is allowed on a low-lectin diet.

Champagne: 3

Possibly fairly high in lectins. However as a rare treat may be okay. For example, Dr Steven Gundry permits drinking champagne occasionally. However we would not recommend making this a regular part of your low-lectin diet.

Chard: 5

Also known as *swiss chard*, these are thought to be low in lectins. However chard is very high in oxalates.

Cheddar cheese: 1

It's thought that cheddar cheese is the *"most concentrated form of casein in any food"* and given that cheeses high in casein proteins are high in lectins, avoid.

Cheese made from unpasteurized "raw" milk: 3

Raw milk cheese include Camembert, Brie, Roquefort, Blue, Washed Rinds etc. (source: Cheese Grotto). Lectin content depends on the type of soft cheese. For example, it's thought that Brie is high in lectins. Test carefully.

Cheeses: 3

Cheeses tend to vary considerably.

It's thought that cheeses high in casein proteins such as Cheddar, Brie, Gouda and Edam are high in lectins.

Certain cheeses acquire lectins from the moulds that grow within it for example, blue cheese (source: *Understanding Arthritis, The Clinical Way Forward by W. Fox, D. Freed*).

Goat and sheep cheeses are acceptable on a low-lectin diet.

However, some source suggest that consuming dairy products such as cheese increases inflammation so it should be avoided altogether.

On the other hand, a study confirmed *"the ability of dairy products to modulate inflammatory processes in humans is an important but unresolved issue"* and *"future research should thus better combine food and nutritional sciences to adequately follow the fate of these nutrients along the gastrointestinal and metabolic axes"*. It therefore seems that more research is needed before concluding whether cheese should be be avoided. Test carefully.

(source: *Bordoni A, Danesi F, Dardevet D, Dupont D, Fernandez AS, Gille D, Nunes Dos Santos C, Pinto P, Re R, Rémond D, Shahar DR, Vergères G. Dairy products and inflammation: A review of the clinical evidence*).

Cherry: 5

Cherries are thought to be low lectin.

Chia, chia seeds: 1

High in lectins. One to put in your 'avoid' list.

Soaking the chia seeds helps reduce lectin content. Why not try basil seeds? These are seeds of basil plants which are edible and similar to chia seeds, they become gelatinous when added to liquid. Basil seeds are a great lectin free alternative.

Chicken: 5

Multiple sources confirm that chicken may be consumed on a low-lectin diet. Avoid corn-fed chicken and opt for pasture-raised chicken.

Chickpeas: 1

High in lectins. One to put in your 'avoid' list.

Chicory: 5

Thought to be low lectin.

Chili pepper, red, fresh: 1

High in lectins. One to put in your 'avoid' list. They are a part of the nightshade family which are high in lectins particularly in the seeds and peels.

To reduce lectin content, Precision Nutrition recommends to peel and de-seed chili peppers before cooking. This is because the highest concentration of lectins can be found in the seeds of plants (source: Diagnosis Diet).

Chives: 5

Thought to be low lectin.

Chocolate: 4

Chocolate is made from fermented cocoa beans. A study found the fermentation process reduces lower lectin content (source: *Sá AGA, Moreno YMF, Carciofi BAM. Food processing for the improvement of plant proteins digestibility*).

Chocolate does contain lectins but these aren't 'toxic lectins' which means the lectins present do not harm the gut barrier (source: Paleo in the UK).

Due to the sugar content in chocolate, we recommend 85-90% cocoa solids as these contain little sugar.

Cilantro: 5

Also known as *coriander*. Thought to be low-lectin.

Cinnamon: 5

Allowed on a low-lectin diet.

Citrus fruits: 3

These include lemons, limes and oranges which are thought to contain some lectins to varying degrees.

Opinion is split with oranges. One source confirmed that oranges are a source of lectins however, another source noted oranges contain D-Mannose, a powerful natural lectin-blocker.

The lectin content varies depending on the fruit but as citrus fruits are high in antioxidants, the benefits outweighs the negatives. It's thought that these could be enjoyed in moderation.

Test carefully, and find more information under individual ingredients.

Clover: 1

A part of the pea family. A study found a pea lectin gene in the roots of white clover (source: *Sugar-Binding Activity of Pea*

Lectin Expressed in White Clover Hairy Roots by Clara L. Díaz, Trudy J. J. Logman, Hanneke C. Stam and Jan W. Kijne). Best to avoid.

Cloves: 5

Thought to be allowed on a low-lectin diet (source: Daytona Wellness Center).

Cocoa butter and cacao butter: 4

Cocoa butter is fat extracted from the cocoa bean. Thought to be low-lectin. As chocolate can be high in sugar content, we recommends 85-90% cocoa solids as these are lower sugar and may represent a healthier choice.

Cocoa drinks, powder, etc: 4

Chocolate does contain lectins but these aren't 'toxic lectins' which means the lectins present in chocolate doesn't harm the gut barrier (source: Paleo in the UK).

As reiterated above, a higher cocoa solids percentage can lead to a lower sugar and potentially healthier option.

Coconut and coconut derivatives: 5

Thought to be low-lectin.

Coffee: 3

Coffee is important! But it is one of those ingredients where opinion is split.

Some of our research has shown coffee contains lectins but as these aren't 'toxic lectins', the lectins present in coffee doesn't harm the gut barrier so it's ok to consume.

Others believe raw coffee beans are high in lectins but since the beans are heated, drinking coffee is safe.

And then there is yet more opinion, including a school of thought which suggests coffee should be avoided altogether.

So who to believe? The major lists disagree considerably, and you should test carefully.

This is one of the reasons we wrote this book, so we could reflect all of the different points of view for you and you can make your own mind up.

Coriander: 5

Also known as *cilantro*. Thought to be low-lectin.

Cornflakes: 1

High in lectins. One to put in your 'avoid' list.

Courgette: 2

Also known as *zucchini*. Mixed opinion. Some sources say these are high in lectin whereas some say it's ok to consume.

Thankfully there are some measures that it is believed will help with lectin content. Peeling and de-seeding is believed to reduce lectin content. Test carefully.

Crab: 5

Thought to be low-lectin.

Crab shells contain high levels of glucosamine (a natural compound found in cartilage)? In fact, glucosamine supplements are often made from lobster, shrimps, crabs and crawfish shells. Next time, don't throw the shells away. Grind them up and sprinkle them over food (source: Human Food Bar).

Cranberries and cranberry juice: 5

We recommend cranberry on a low lectin diet. It's a great option and may even help you lower your lectin levels.

Health Canal's website refers to cranberry as a "natural lectin blocker" as it binds lectins and helps the body absorb them more efficiently.

Crawfish: 1

Also known as *crayfish*. Avoid crayfish as lectins have been found in freshwater crayfish (source: *Zhang XW, Wang XW, Sun C, Zhao XF, Wang JX. C-type lectin from red swamp crayfish Procambarus clarkii participates in cellular immune response.*)

Crayfish: 1

Also known as *crawfish*. Avoid crayfish as lectins have been found in freshwater crayfish (source: *Zhang XW, Wang XW, Sun C, Zhao XF, Wang JX. C-type lectin from red swamp crayfish Procambarus clarkii participates in cellular immune response.*)

Cream cheeses: 3

Some sources claim that very high fat dairy products such as cream cheeses are low in casein and therefore low in lectin. Other sources mention all dairy products contain casein and should be avoided. Test carefully.

Cream: 3

As above, some sources claim that very high fat dairy products such as cream are low in casein and therefore low in lectin. Other sources mention all dairy products contain casein and should be avoided. Test carefully.

Cress: 3

Thought to contain some lectins. Test carefully.

Cucumber: 2

Mixed opinion. Precision Nutrition recommends to peel and de-seed cucumbers before cooking to reduce lectin content. This is because the highest concentration of lectins can be found in the seeds of plants (source: Diagnosis Diet).

However, Kimberly Gomer, Director of Nutrition at the Pritikin Longevity Center in Miami confirmed the lectins found in cucumber "whether cooked or consumed raw, do not appear to cause significant GI problems". Test carefully.

Cumin: 4

After careful analysis we've found limited research on cumin and lectins. Since dill is a part of the Apiaceae family (which includes parsley, parsnip, celery and carrot), cumin could be allowed on a low-lectin diet.

Curry: 4

Depends on the ingredients in the curry. The most common ingredients are thought to include garlic, ginger, turmeric, black pepper and onions to name a few which are allowed on a low-lectin diet.

Dates: 3

Moderate lectin content. Test carefully.

Dextrose: 1

Sugar from corn. We know that all corn-foods should be avoided. Opt for honey as an alternative to sugar.

Dill: 4

Since dill is a part of the Apiaceae family (which includes parsley, parsnip, celery and carrot), dill could be allowed on a low-lectin diet.

Dragon fruit: 3

Often known as white-fleshed pitahaya. Dragon fruits are an excellent source of fiber, magnesium, iron, vitamin C, carotenoids and lycopene. It seems that this fruit may be enjoyed as part of a healthy diet. Test carefully.

Dried fruit: 3

We think the lectin content depends on the type of dried fruit but it's unclear whether the drying process reduces lectin content. Test carefully.

A great snack but watch the sugar content. The drying process removes water from the fruit but this means a higher concentration of sugar (source: New York Times).

Dried meat: 5

Includes grass-fed jerky which is allowed on a low-lectin diet. Ensure these are grass-fed.

Dry-cured meats: 5

These are meats that have been salted, dried and aged to preserve them from harmful bacteria. Dry-cured meats Include jamon, prosciutto and salami etc.

As meats are generally low in lectins, dry-cured meats are allowed on a low-lectin diet. Ensure these are grass-fed.

Duck: 5

Allowed on a low-lectin diet. Opt for pasture-raised duck.

Egg white: 3

Depends on the type of egg. Always buy pasture-raised eggs as these contain the least amount of lectins.

According to Lectin Free Mama's blog, "duck eggs make fluffier, higher-raised baking goods than chicken eggs". Why not try baking with duck eggs?

Egg yolk: 3

Depends on the type of egg. Always buy pasture-raised eggs as these contain the least amount of lectins.

Elderflower cordial: 2

Elderflower contains lectins and it's thought to come from the same tree as elderberries. A study found lectins present in the barks of elderberries (source: *Nsimba-Lubaki M, Peumans WJ. Seasonal Fluctuations of Lectins in Barks of Elderberry (Sambucus nigra) and Black Locust (Robinia pseudoacacia)*) Test carefully.

Endive: 5

Allowed on a low-lectin diet.

Espresso: 4

Coffee is one of those ones where opinion is split. Some say coffee does contain lectins but as these aren't 'toxic lectins', the lectins present in coffee doesn't harm the gut barrier so it's ok to consume.

Others say raw coffee beans are high in lectins but since the beans are heated, drinking coffee is safe. On the other hand, some argue that coffee should be avoided altogether. Test carefully.

Fennel: 5

Allowed on a low-lectin diet.

Fenugreek: 3

There are lectins present in fenugreek (source: Food and Nutrition Journal). Test carefully.

Feta cheese: 3

Thought to be low-lectin if made with sheep or goat milk. Traditional feta cheese is made with sheep or goat milk but nowadays, cow's milk is also used.

Check before consuming.

Figs (fresh or dried): 5

These are actually flowers and not a fruit! Thought to be low-lectin.

Fish: 3

Depends on the type. Check individual fish in this list.

Whitefish are lobsters and thought to be low in lectins.

Avoid crayfish as lectins have been found in freshwater crayfish (source: *Zhang XW, Wang XW, Sun C, Zhao XF, Wang JX. C-type lectin from red swamp crayfish Procambarus clarkii participates in cellular immune response*).

Lectins were also reported in trout (source: *Ng TB, Fai Cheung RC, Wing Ng CC, Fang EF, Wong JH. A review of fish lectins*).

Flaxseed (linseed): 5

Allowed on a low-lectin diet.

Fructose (fruit sugar): 2

According to the RDH (Registered Dental Hygienists), there is no biological need for fructose. RDH lists the negative health implications of consuming fructose such as the increase risk of obesity and type 2 diabetes to name a few.

It's unclear whether fructose contains lectins but due to the potential negative health implications, we recommend avoiding processed fructose where possible. However, there are foods naturally high in fructose such as apples, pears and honey which are allowed on a low lectin diet. These may be consumed in moderation.

Game (meat): 5

Allowed on a low-lectin diet. Opt for pasture-raised game.

Garlic: 5

Garlic falls under the lowest lectin content options for a low-lectin diet .

Ginger: 5

Allowed on a low-lectin diet.

Goat's milk: 5

Goat's milk contains much less/no A1 beta-casein protein compared to cow's milk which means they are allowed on a low-lectin diet.

Goji berry: 1

A part of the nightshade family which are high in lectins.

Goose (organic, freshly cooked): 5

Allowed on a low-lectin diet. Opt for pasture-raised goose.

Gooseberry, gooseberries: 2

Not a lot of information out there but since gooseberries are related to currants, we think they could also be a source of lectins. Test carefully.

Gouda cheese: 1

Avoid. It's thought that Gouda cheese is made from casein proteins which are high in lectins.

Grapefruit: 3

Moderate lectin content but given the high antioxidants and enormous health benefits, these can be enjoyed in moderation.

Grapes: 3

Moderate lectin content. Limit grape consumption due to their high sugar levels.

Note that the nutrition content of grapes depend on how they're grown. For example, it's thought that grapes grown at a higher altitude have more exposure to the sun so they contain higher levels of Polyphenols (anti-oxidants) (source: Katherine Senko: Polyphenols in Wine).

Green beans: 1

High in lectins. One to put in your 'avoid' list.

If you want to consume beans, the FDA recommends boiling them for 30 minutes to reduce lectin content.

Avoid canned beans as most of these haven't been soaked or cooked to reduce lectin content.

Green peas: 3

Mixed opinion. Some say they contain low levels of lectins and are safe to eat. However, others believe they may interfere with gut absorption.

A study found that soaking peas *"significantly decreased the contents of lectins"* (source: *Shi L, Arntfield SD, Nickerson M. Changes in levels of phytic acid, lectins and oxalates during soaking and cooking of Canadian pulses*).

Limit consumption and test carefully initially.

Green tea: 4

It's thought that tea is allowed on a low-lectin diet. A study found that green tea *"can be beneficial for people exposed to plant lectins"* as it *"alleviates hepatic inflammatory damage and immunological reaction"* in mice. The green tea polyphenols (antioxidants) *"exert protective effects"*

(source: *Wang D, Zhang M, Wang T, Liu T, Guo Y, Granato D. Green tea polyphenols mitigate the plant lectins-induced liver inflammation and immunological reaction in C57BL/6 mice via NLRP3 and Nrf2 signaling pathways*)

Guava: 3

Thought to contain moderate lectins.

Ham (dried, cured): 5

Allowed on a low-lectin diet. Ensure these are grass-fed.

Hazelnut: 5

Allowed on a low-lectin diet. A great alternative to peanuts.

Hemp seeds (Cannabis sativa): 5

Seeds usually contain lectins but not hemp seeds. These are thought to be very low or free of lectins

Herbal tea: 5

It's thought that tea is allowed on a low-lectin diet.

Honey: 5

Allowed on a low-lectin diet however, note the high sugar content. Consume in moderation.

Horseradish: 5

Falls under the cruciferous vegetable family (includes broccoli, kale, cabbage, radish etc.). These are thought to be low-lectin and rich in vitamin C, folate and fiber.

Juniper berries: 3

Don't be confused by it's name, despite looking like blueberries these aren't consumed like berries due to the bitterness.

Used as a bitter spice for a range of dishes, we know that spices may be consumed on a low-lectin diet so perhaps these may also be allowed.

Kale: 5

Falls under the cruciferous vegetable family (includes broccoli, Brussel sprouts, cabbage, radish etc.). These are thought to be low-lectin and rich in vitamin C, folate and fiber.

Kefir: 1

Avoid. Contains A1 casein protein.

Kelp: 5

Thought to be low-lectin.

Kiwi: 5

Health Canal's website refers to kiwi as a "natural lectin blocker" because kiwi increases the production of mucin in our bodies. Mucin contains sialic acid which blocks lectins from causing harm to our digestive system. Best to consume when kiwi is in season.

Kohlrabi: 5

Thought to be low-lectin.

Lamb: 5

Allowed on a low-lectin diet. Opt for grass-fed lamb.

Lamb's lettuce, corn salad: 1

Corn Salad is made with corn kernels and all corn-foods should be avoided.

Lard: 5

A low-lectin fat made of 100% pork fat.

Leek: 4

Contains little lectin. Test carefully.

Lemon: 3

These are a source of lectins but given the high antioxidants, the benefits outweighs the negatives. It's thought that these can be enjoyed in moderation. Test carefully.

Lentils: 1

High in lectins. Lentils are thought to be especially high in lectins.

Lettuce: 5

Thought to be low-lectin.

Lime: 3

These are a source of lectins but given the high antioxidants, the benefits outweighs the negatives. It's thought that these can be enjoyed in moderation. Test carefully.

Liquor: 3

Aged liquors are acceptable on a low-lectin diet.

Liquorice: 3

Also known as *licorice*. One source mentioned that supplements containing liquorice root helps to heal a leaky gut. Another source mentioned that liquorice contains concentrated levels of lectins. Test carefully.

Avoid large quantities of liquorice as this could contribute to increase in blood pressure and arrhythmia (source: NHS).

Lobster: 5

Thought to be low in lectin.

Loganberry: 3

A cross between raspberries and blackberries. As raspberries and blackberries are thought to contain moderate amounts of lectins, we think that loganberry should be rated the same.

Lychee: 2

Also known as *litchi*. A study found lectins in the seeds of litchi fruits (source: *A glucose/mannose binding lectin from litchi (Litchi chinensis) seeds: Biochemical and biophysical characterizations*). Test carefully.

According to the US Department of Agriculture, a cup of lychees contains almost 29g of sugar. We therefore suggest limiting lychee consumption. If choosing canned lychees, go for water-packed canned lychees and check the sugar content and avoid those with added sweeteners.

Never consume unripe lychees. These are poisonous and can cause extremely low blood sugar (source: CNN Health).

Macadamia: 5

Allowed on a low-lectin diet.

Malt extract: 1

Derived from barley grains. Avoid as barley is high in lectins.

Malt: 1

Avoid barley malt as barley is high in lectins.

Maltodextrin: 1

Used to thicken foods and liquids, improve texture, flavour and increase shelf life, maltodextrin has no nutritional value (source: Medical News Today). It's also highly processed and high in lectins.

Not an ingredient we like. One to put in your 'avoid' list.

Mandarin orange: 3

Opinion is split. One source confirmed that oranges are a source of lectins however, another source noted oranges contain D-Mannose, a powerful natural lectin-blocker. Test carefully.

Mango: 5

Allowed on a low lectin diet however, we believe a lower sugar diet is better for overall health, therefore consumption of ripe mangoes due to their high sugar levels.

Maple syrup: 1

Due to the higher sugar content, maple syrup should be avoided. Yacon syrup has been recommended instead.

Margarine: 1

A processed food - thought to be high in lectins.

Marrow: 2

This is a courgette that has been left to grow for longer. Thought to be a source of lectins, as are courgettes (see courgette). Removing the seeds may help lower the lectin content, and this is easier with a marrow than a courgette.

Mascarpone cheese: 3

A type of soft Italian cream cheese. Some sources claim that very high fat dairy products such as cream cheeses are low in casein and therefore low in lectin. Other sources mention all dairy products contain casein and should be avoided. Test carefully.

Mate tea: 5

It's thought that tea is allowed on a low-lectin diet.

Melon: 1

High in lectins. One to put in your 'avoid' list.

Milk: 3

Goat and sheep milk are acceptable on a low-lectin diet.

As for cow's milk. It depends on the type. Certain milks are high in A1 casein which can be high in lectins.

It's thought that milk from cows that originate in the Channel Islands and Southern France are better on a low-lectin diet. Test store bought milk carefully.

Millet: 5

A lectin-free grain and high in anti-oxidants. Allowed on a low-lectin diet.

Minced meat: 5

Avoid corn-fed minced meat and opt for grass-fed instead.

Mint: 5

Thought to be low-lectin.

Morel: 5

A type of wild mushroom that's difficult to find (source: Wild Food UK). As these are rare, they tend to be expensive and used in gourmet meals.

Given that most mushrooms contain relatively low lectin, morels should be the same too.

Morello cherries: 4

A type of sour cherry. Given that morello cherries are a type of cherry, it should be low in lectins. Test carefully.

Mozzarella cheese: 3

Mozzarella is thought to contain less casein protein than hard cheeses. Test carefully.

Mulberry: 1

A rich source of lectins (source: *Saeed B, Baranwal VK, Khurana P. Identification and Expression Profiling of the Lectin Gene Superfamily in Mulberry*). One to put in your 'avoid' list.

Mung beans (germinated, sprouting): 2

A source of lectins although lectin content is reduced significantly after the sprouting process (source: Superfood Evolution). Sprouting can be done at home by following the below process:

"1) Soak legumes to soften, 2) rinse well with cool water, 3) drain water from jar 4) Repeat steps 2 and 3 until sprouts form and 5) Store in the fridge until ready to eat." (source: *Live Eat Learn*)

Avoid consuming mung bean sprouts raw.

Mushrooms, different types: 5

Mushrooms fall under the lowest lectin content options for a low-lectin diet.

Mustard and mustard seeds: 5

Allowed on a low-lectin diet.

Napa cabbage: 5

Also known as *Chinese Cabbage*. Falls under the cruciferous vegetable family (includes broccoli, kale, Brussel sprouts, radish etc.). These are thought to be low-lectin and rich in vitamin C, folate and fiber.

Nectarine: 5

Best to consume when nectarine is in season. As with other fruits, when in season it may contain less lectins than when they're out of season.

Nettle tea: 1

A study found "unusual" lectins in stinging nettles (source: *Science Direct: An unusual lectin from stinging nettle (Urtica dioica) rhizomes*). Best to avoid.

Nori seaweed: 5

Allowed on a low-lectin diet.

Nutmeg: 3

Contains some lectins. Test carefully.

Nuts: 3

Depends on the type of nut. For example, cashew and peanuts are high in lectins.

Check individual nuts in this food list.

Oats: 1

Oats are considered to be high in lectins and a major culprit for those on a low lectin diet.

Consider sprouted oats instead as these contain less lectins and should digest better. The sprouting process is thought to reduce the lectin content and make them more easy to digest.

Also it's thought by some that cooking oats also reduces the lectin content.

Olive oil: 4

A source confirms that olive oil is allowed on the lectin-free diet. The Woodland Institute notes that olive oil contains some lectins but as they're full of antioxidants and healthy monounsaturated fats, the benefits outweighs the negatives. It's thought that they can be eaten without restriction and it's not necessary to eliminate them from your diet. Test carefully.

Human Food Bar's website mention *"the benefits of olive oil very greatly depending on how the olives are sourced and oil is made"*. For example, vacuum-extracted olive oil is thought to be better as the process reduces exposure to oxygen and retains polyphenols (anti-oxidants) (source: Apollo Olive Oil).

As extra extra-virgin olive oil is the least processed form of olive oil, opt for vacuum-extracted extra-virgin olive oil.

Olives: 4

As per olive oil, olives contains some lectins but as they're full of antioxidants and healthy monounsaturated fats, the benefits outweigh the negatives. It's thought that they can be eaten without restriction and it's not necessary to eliminate them from your diet. Test carefully.

Onion: 5

Onions fall under the lowest lectin content options for a low lectin diet.

Orange: 3

Opinion is split. One source confirmed that oranges are a source of lectins however, another source noted oranges contain D-Mannose, a powerful natural lectin-blocker. Test carefully.

Oregano: 2

Contains some lectins. Obviously depends on quantities used.

Dr Suzanne Joy S Stuart of Naturally Balanced Health recommends limiting or avoiding oregano.

Ostrich: 5

Not admittedly, a particularly common food but it still makes it into our food list. Fine on a low-lectin diet.

Opt for pasture-raised meat when possible.

Oyster: 5

Full of health benefits. Oysters are high in protein, vitamin D, zinc, iron and copper (source: Gourmet Food Store) plus they're allowed on a low-lectin diet.

Papaya: 5

Allowed on a low-lectin diet.

However papaya is very high in histamine so those with multiple food sensitivities may want to avoid.

Parsley: 2

Contains some lectins. Dr Suzanne Joy S Stuart of Naturally Balanced Health recommends limiting or avoiding oregano.

Parsnip: 5

Allowed on a low-lectin diet. This is an effective alternative to potato (which is high in lectins. One to put in your 'avoid' list).

Passion fruit: 5

Allowed on a low-lectin diet. Consume when passion fruit is in-season.

Pasta: 2

The short answer is it depends what the pasta is made from.

Wheat flour contains a lectin called wheat germ agglutinin (WGA). A study found variable amounts of WGA in wholemeal pasta *"probably as a consequence of thermal inactivation during food processing"* (source: *Temperature-dependent decay of wheat germ agglutinin activity and its implications for food processing and analysis*). It seems that cooking reduces lectin content.

Opt for whole-wheat pasta. Another study found:

"*Commercial pasta products labeled as whole wheat were also tested for WGA content and found to contain up to 90% less WGA compared to a whole grain standard.*"

(source: *Killilea DW, McQueen R, Abegania JR. Wheat germ agglutinin is a biomarker of whole grain content in wheat flour and pasta.*)

There is also a wide array of non-wheat pastas available and you can check the individual ingredients on this list. For example there are pastas on sale made from almond flour (with skin removed) which may be a better choice on a low-lectin diet.

Peach: 5

Allowed on a low-lectin diet. As with most fruit in our food list, ideally consume when peaches are in season, although this may not always be possible, peaches should still be fine.

Peanuts: 1

High in lectins. It's thought that cooking peanuts may not eliminate their lectin content. Avoid peanuts and also peanut butter.

Pear: 5

Allowed on a low-lectin diet however, note the high sugar content.

Peas (green): 3

Mixed opinion. Some say they contain low levels of lectins and are safe to eat. However, others believe they may interfere with gut absorption.

A study found that soaking peas *"significantly decreased the contents of lectins"* (source: *Shi L, Arntfield SD, Nickerson M. Changes in levels of phytic acid, lectins and oxalates during soaking and cooking of Canadian pulses*).

Limit consumption and test carefully initially.

Pea Shoots (or pea sprouts): 1

There is a slight difference here. Pea sprouts are seeds grown in a jar (without soil) whereas, pea shoots are plants grown in the soil. Seeds are high in lectins so we suggest limiting consumption of pea sprouts. Test pea shoots carefully as these are a part of the pea family.

Peppermint tea: 5

It's thought that tea is allowed on a low-lectin diet.

Pickled food: 5

Allowed on a low-lectin diet.

Pineapple: 5

Allowed on a low-lectin diet however, note the high sugar content.

Pistachio: 3

This is a nut where opinion is mixed, and one of the reasons we wrote this book is because major lists often disagree.

For example, it's thought to be low lectin according to the website Healthline but multiple other research sources show pistachios as containing problematic lectins. Test carefully, and we will update this list as new research becomes available.

Plum: 5

Low in lectins.

Pomegranate: 5

Allowed on a low-lectin diet. Loaded with vitamin C and also low in histamines for those watching out for multiple food sensitivities.

Poppy seeds: 1

High in lectins. One to put in your 'avoid' list.

Pork: 5

Allowed on a low-lectin diet. Opt for grass-fed meat for a much healthier dish.

Potato: 1

Potatoes are high in lectins.

Although cooking reduces lectin content, it's thought that potato lectins are quite resistant and will only reduce by 50-60% (source: The Woodlands Institute for health and wellness).

Poultry meat: 5

Allowed on a low-lectin diet. Opt for pastured poultry meat.

Prawn: 2

Closely related to shrimp, many believe these could also be a source of lectins.

Processed cheese: 2

Cheese mixed with artificial ingredients such as flavour enhancers, colouring etc. so that it can no longer be classified as cheese. These also contain 2-3 times more sodium than unprocessed cheese (source: Ricardo Cuisine).

The lectin content depends on the type of cheese used in the process but given that these aren't as healthy as regular cheese, we recommend limiting consumption of processed cheese.

If consuming processed cheese, opt for cheese produced from A2 milk (from cows that originate in the Channel Islands and Southern France). Easier said than done we know. Knowing the type of milk used during cheese production will help you assess. Test carefully.

Prune: 5

A dried plum. As plums are low in lectin content, it's thought that it's allowed on a low lectin diet.

Pulses: 1

Include beans, peas and lentils which are all high in lectins to varying degrees.

Check individual ingredients.

Pumpkin seed oil: 1

High in lectins.

Pumpkin seeds: 1

High in lectins.

To reduce lectin content, Precision Nutrition recommends soaking and cooking pumpkin seeds. This is because the highest concentration of lectins can be found in the seeds of plants (source: Diagnosis Diet).

Pumpkin: 1

Pumpkin is a source of lectins (source: Functional Nutrition Library). Peeling and de-seeding helps to reduce lectin content.

Quinoa: 1

High in lectins. One to put in your 'avoid' list.

Rabbit: 5

Thought to be low-lectin. Opt for grass-fed rabbit.

Raclette cheese: 4

A traditional Swiss melting cheese. It seems that most cheese from Switzerland is produced from A2 cow's milk (cows that originate in the Channel Islands and Southern France). If this is the case with raclette cheese then it's thought to be allowed on a low lectin diet.

Radish: 5

Falls under the cruciferous vegetable family (includes broccoli, kale, cabbage, radish etc.). These are thought to be low lectin and rich in vitamin C, folate and fiber.

Raisins: 3

Raisins are dried grapes and we know that grapes contain moderate lectin content. Consume in moderation due to high sugar content.

Note that the nutrition content of grapes depend on how they are grown. For example, it's thought that grapes grown at a higher altitude are exposed to the sun so they contain higher levels of Polyphenols (anti-oxidants) (source: Katherine Senko: Polyphenols in Wine).

Rapeseed oil (called canola oil in US): 1

High in lectins. One to put in your 'avoid' list.

Raspberry: 4

Contains relatively low-lectins.

Scores a 4 not a 5 on our food list but should be reasonably acceptable on a low-lectin diet in moderate quantities.

Red cabbage: 5

One of the cabbage varieties, thought to be low-lectin.

Red wine vinegar: 5

It's thought that all types of vinegar are allowed on a low-lectin diet.

Redcurrants: 2

A member of the gooseberry family. As studies on redcurrants and lectins are limited, we recommend proceeding with caution. Since gooseberries are related to currants, we think they could also be a source of lectins.

Rhubarb: 4

Contains very little lectin. Consuming shouldn't cause any issues but test carefully.

Rice: 1

Mixed opinion. One source points to no lectins in rice however, a study found lectins in rice (source: *Al Atalah B, De Vleesschauwer D, Xu J, Fouquaert E, Höfte M, Van Damme EJ. Transcriptional behavior of EUL-related rice lectins toward important abiotic and biotic stresses*).

Other sources confirm that white rice contains fewer lectins than brown rice. It's recommended to use a pressure cooker to kill off lectins. It's thought that boiling rice also reduces lectin content.

Best to avoid.

Rice cakes: 1

A snack food made from puffed rice. As above, there is mixed opinion on the consumption of rice. Best to avoid.

Rice milk: 1

Milk made from rice. As above, there is mixed opinion on the consumption of rice. Test carefully.

Watch out for added ingredients in rice milks. As a rule of thumb, the fewer ingredients, the better.

Rice noodles: 1

Made from rice flour which are high in lectins. Best to avoid.

Ricotta cheese: 3

Depends on the milk as ricotta cheese can be made from cow, sheep, goat or water buffalo's milk (source: Bon Appetit). Avoid ricotta cheese made from cow's milk.

Rooibos tea: 5

It's thought that tea is allowed on a low-lectin diet.

Roquefort cheese: 3

A type of blue cheese made from sheep's milk. Cheese acquires lectins from the moulds that grow within it (source: *Understanding Arthritis, The Clinical Way Forward by W. Fox, D. Freed*). Test carefully as moulds are used in roquefort production.

Rosemary: 5

Allowed on a low-lectin diet.

Rum: 3

A distilled spirit made from fermented sugar (source: Vine Pair). As studies on rum and lectins are limited, we recommend proceeding with caution.

Rye: 1

A cereal grain high in lectins. One to put in your 'avoid' list. Avoid foods containing rye such as rye bread, crackers, beer and whiskey (source: The Spruce Eats).

Sage: 5

Allowed on a low-lectin diet.

Salami: 5

A cured sausage. As meats are generally low in lectins, dry-cured meats such as salami are allowed on a low-lectin diet. Ensure the salami is made from grass-fed meat.

Salmon: 5

Allowed on a low-lectin diet. For a healthier option, opt for wild caught salmon. These are lower in calories and have higher levels of potassium and other minerals (source: Wild For Salmon).

Sauerkraut: 5

Raw sauerkraut is thought to be low-lectin.

Sausages of all kinds: 5

Fresh sausages without high lectin ingredients are allowed (source: US Wellness Meats). Opt for grass-fed sausages.

Sausages can have other, added ingredients, so check carefully.

Savoy cabbage: 5

One of the cabbage varieties, thought to be low-lectin.

Schnapps: 3

As studies on schnapps (a type of alcohol) and lectins are limited, we recommend proceeding with caution.

Seafood: 3

Depends on the type. Wild-caught seafood is thought to be low in lectin.

Seaweed: 5

Thought to be low-lectin. Health Canal's website refers to bladderwrack seaweed as a "natural lectin blocker".

Sesame: 1

Sesame is a source of lectins (source: Functional Nutrition Library).

Sheep's milk, sheep milk: 5

Allowed on a low-lectin diet.

Importantly, sheep milk is often digested easier than normal dairy as it contains more A2 beta-casein proteins (source: Parsley Health).

Shellfish: 2

A source of lectins. One to put in your 'avoid' list (source: *Live Pain Free Cookbook by Jesse Cannone*).

Shrimp: 1

Seven groups of lectins have been found in shrimp (source: *Wang XW, Wang JX. Diversity and multiple functions of lectins in shrimp immunity. Dev Comp Immunol*).

While we have not found a conclusive answer to the shrimp content in lectin, we believe it is best to avoid or approach with caution.

Smoked fish: 5

If wild caught then allowed on a low-lectin diet.

Smoked meat: 5

Allowed but ensure these are grass-fed.

Snow peas: 3

Also known as *Chinese pea pods*.

Mixed opinion. Some say these contain low levels of lectin and are safe to eat.

However, Dr Cordain mentioned on The Paleo Diet's website that consuming peas *"may still interfere with normal gut nutrient absorption"*.

Limit consumption and test carefully.

Soft cheese: 3

Soft cheese typically includes feta, brie, ricotta, cream cheese, mozzarella and cottage cheese to name a few. Lectin content depends on the type of soft cheese. For example, Feta is thought to be low-lectin if made with sheep or goat milk and cottage cheese should be avoided according to some sources.

Note that some sources claim that very high fat dairy products such as soft cheeses are low in casein and therefore low in lectin. Other sources mention all dairy products contain casein and should be avoided. Test carefully.

Sour cream: 3

Some sources claim that very high fat dairy products such as sour cream are low in casein and therefore low in lectin. Other sources mention all dairy products contain casein and should be avoided. Test carefully.

Soy (soy beans, soy flour): 1

Soy beans are high in lectins. One to put in your 'avoid' list.

According to the Food Chemistry Journal Volume 39, Issue 3, 1991, the amount of lectin in soy flour depends on the processing method used. Soy flour made from raw seeds contained the highest level of lectins.

Successful attempts have been made to remove lectins from soybean flour using a bio-separation technique (source: *S. Bajpai et al. / Food Chemistry 89 (2005) 497-501*) but as these techniques cannot easily be performed in the kitchen, it's best to avoid.

Soy sauce: 1

High in lectins. One to put in your 'avoid' list. See soy above.

Sparkling wine: 3

Lectin content should depend on the type of sparkling wine. Test carefully.

We know that red wine contains high levels of Polyphenols (antioxidants) compared to other types of wine (including white wine). Some experts permit drinking wine high in Polyphenols (in moderation) on a low-lectin diet.

Note that the nutrition content of red wine depend on how the grapes are grown. For example, it's thought that grapes grown at a higher altitude have a greater exposure to the sun so they contain higher levels of Polyphenols (source: Katherine Senko: Polyphenols in Wine).

Spelt: 1

A type of grain. Grains are high in lectins. Avoid.

Spinach: 5

Thought to be low-lectin. Spinach is extremely high in oxalate and relatively high in histamine so one to avoid for those with multiple food sensitivities.

Spirits: 3

As studies on spirits and lectins are limited, we recommend proceeding with caution. See 'alcohol' for more on spirits and lectins.

Squashes: 2

Thought to be high in lectin. Peeling and de-seeding helps to reduce lectin content.

Stevia: 4

A great alternative to sugar. Allowed on a low-lectin diet.

Stinging nettle: 1

A study found "unusual" lectins in stinging nettles (source: *Science Direct: An unusual lectin from stinging nettle (Urtica dioica) rhizomes*). Best to avoid.

Strawberry: 5

Contains relatively low lectins.

Sugar: 1

Avoid. While we realise that is easier said than done, sugar is not actually required in your diet and consuming too much can raise blood pressure (source: Havard Health). Opt for honey as an alternative to sugar - but still use in moderation.

Sunflower oil: 1

High in lectins. One to put in your 'avoid' list.

Sunflower seeds: 1

High in lectins. To reduce lectin content, Precision Nutrition recommends soaking and cooking sunflower seeds. This is because the highest concentration of lectins can be found in the seeds of plants (source: Diagnosis Diet).

Sweetcorn: 1

Also known as *corn on the cob*. High in lectins.

Corn is very resistant to heat therefore, it's hard to reduce the lectin content.

Sweet potato: 4

Unlike white potatoes, sweet potatoes are thought to be low in lectins and high in anti-oxidants.

A much better source for your potato needs on a low-lectin diet.

Tea, black: 5

It's thought that tea is allowed on a low-lectin diet.

Thyme: 4

Allowed on a low-lectin diet.

Tomato: 1

High in lectins. One to put in your 'avoid' list. They're a part of the nightshade family which are thought to be high in lectins particularly in the seeds and peels.

Precision Nutrition recommends something rather fiddly, but potentially helpful. It suggests to peel and de-seed tomatoes before cooking to reduce lectin content. This is because the highest concentration of lectins can be found in the seeds of plants (source: Diagnosis Diet).

Trout: 2

A study found lectins reported in trout (source: *Ng TB, Fai Cheung RC, Wing Ng CC, Fang EF, Wong JH. A review of fish lectins*) although we're unclear on the amount of lectins and whether these are harmful.

Trout and salmon are closely related as they belong to the same fish family (source The Kitchen Community). Salmon is allowed on a low lectin diet so it could be that trout is allowed too. Test carefully.

Tuna: 5

Low in lectins. For a healthier option, opt for wild caught tuna. These are thought to be less contaminated from man-made toxins as the fish feed on a natural diet (source: The Nest).

Often thought to be high in mercury so eat rarely.

Turkey: 5

Allowed on a low-lectin diet. Opt for pasture-raised turkey.

Turmeric: 5

Packed with anti-oxidants and allowed on a low-lectin diet.

Turnip: 5

Falls under the cruciferous vegetable family (includes broccoli, kale, cabbage, radish etc.). These are thought to be low lectin and rich in vitamin C, folate and fiber.

Vanilla: 5

Allowed on a low-lectin diet.

Venison: 5

Meat from the deer. Allowed on a low-lectin diet. Opt for grass-fed venison.

Vinegar: balsamic: 5

It's thought that all types of vinegar are allowed on a low-lectin diet.

Vinegar: distilled white vinegar: 5

It's thought that all types of vinegar are allowed on a low-lectin diet.

Walnut: 3

Mixed opinion. Some sources point to walnuts being allowed on a low-lectin diet whereas, another source noted that walnuts contain lectins. Test carefully.

Watercress: 5

Falls under the cruciferous vegetable family (includes broccoli, kale, cabbage, radish etc.). These are thought to be low-lectin and rich in vitamin C, folate and fiber.

Watermelon: 2

Thought to contain high amounts of lectins.

Wheat: 1

Wheat is considered to be a grain of the seed (source: Diagnosis Diet). Grains are considered high in lectins and should be avoided. Look for gluten-free alternatives and check ingredients.

Wheat germ: 1

The germ of a cereal and part of a wheat kernel. As wheat is considered to be a grain of the seed, we know that grains are high in lectins. Avoid.

White button mushroom: 5

Mushrooms fall under the lowest lectin content options for a low-lectin diet.

Wild rice: 2

Not actually a rice - it's an aquatic grass (fun fact). Wild rice requires to be cooked for longer than white and brown rice (source: The Spruce Eats). It's thought that using a pressure cooker and boiling rice reduces lectin content. Test carefully.

Wine: 3

It seems that dessert wines, sweet wines and white wines should be avoided. Given the high sugar content, these wines don't seem to have the same benefits as red wine.

Red wine contains high levels of Polyphenols (antioxidants) compared to other types of wine (including white wine). Some experts permit drinking wine high in Polyphenols (in moderation) on a low-lectin diet.

Note that the nutrition content of red wine depend on how the grapes are grown. For example, it's thought that grapes grown at a higher altitude have a greater exposure to the sun so they contain higher levels of Polyphenols (source: Katherine Senko: Polyphenols in Wine).

Yam: 5

Allowed on a low-lectin diet.

Yeast: 1

One to put in your 'avoid' list.

Yogurt/Yoghurt: 3

Produced by fermenting milk and bacteria. A study found the fermentation process reduces lower lectin content (source: *Sá AGA, Moreno YMF, Carciofi BAM. Food processing for the improvement of plant proteins digestibility*).

Be cautious of yogurt made from A1 casein protein and sweetened yogurt.

Goat and sheep yogurt are acceptable on a low-lectin diet. Coconut yogurt may also be a good alternative but please check other ingredients.

Zucchini: 2

Also known as *courgette.* There is mixed opinion on zucchini, but it is generally thought to be high in lectin content.

Peeling and de-seeding helps to reduce lectin content and some sources say it's ok to consume courgette/zucchini. Test carefully.

Made in the USA
Coppell, TX
19 June 2023

18284176R00044